THE KETO CODE

Unlocking the Secrets of Weight Loss and Optimal Health

BY

MISTY JACKSON

Copyright© Misty Jackson

All rights reserved.

TABLE OF CONTENT

Introduction

Chapter 1

Introduction - Cracking the Code

Understanding the Challenges of Weight Loss

Introducing the Ketogenic Lifestyle

Setting the Stage for Success

Chapter 2

Demystifying Ketosis

The Science Behind Ketosis

Benefits of Ketosis for Weight Loss

Beyond Weight Loss & Additional Health Benefits

Understanding the Mechanisms of Ketosis

Chapter 3

The Power of Macronutrients

Understanding Fats, Proteins, and Carbohydrates

Finding the Optimal Macronutrient Ratio for Ketosis

Calculating and Tracking Macros for Success

Chapter 4

Crafting Delicious and Nutritious Keto Meals

Building a Keto-Friendly Pantry

Creating Balanced and Flavorful Keto Meals

Meal Planning and Preparation

Chapter 5
Overcoming Challenges on the Ketogenic Journey

Chapter 6
Optimizing Your Ketogenic Lifestyle

Chapter 7
Sustaining Long-Term Success on the Ketogenic Journey

Chapter 8
Beyond the Ketogenic Lifestyle

Chapter 9
Navigating Challenges and Maintaining Motivation

Chapter 10
Sustaining Long-Term Success Introduction:

Chapter 11
Navigating Social Situations and Maintaining Ketogenic Success

Chapter 12
Overcoming Plateaus and Challenges on the Ketogenic Journey

Chapter 13
Sustaining Long-Term Success on the Ketogenic Journey

Chapter 14
Troubleshooting Common Challenges on the Ketogenic Journey

Chapter 15
Sustainable Ketogenic Living for Long-Term Health

Introduction

In a world saturated with diet trends and conflicting information, it's no wonder that finding a sustainable approach to weight loss and overall well-being can feel like cracking a code.

But fear not, because the key to transforming your body and reclaiming your health lies within these pages.

Imagine a lifestyle where you can indulge in delicious, satisfying meals while shedding unwanted pounds.

Envision a state of vibrant energy and mental clarity that propels you through your days with a renewed sense of purpose.

This is the power of the ketogenic diet—a revolutionary approach to nutrition that has taken the world by storm.

"The Keto Code" is not just another diet book.

It's a comprehensive guide that will empower you to navigate the intricacies of ketosis, understand the science behind it, and unlock the potential for long-term success.

Whether you're a complete beginner or someone who has dabbled in keto before, this book will serve as your roadmap to a healthier, leaner you, Together, we will delve into the fascinating world of ketosis—a metabolic state in which your body switches from using carbohydrates as its primary fuel source to burning fat instead.

By consuming a high-fat, low-carbohydrate diet, you will train your body to become a fat-burning machine, resulting in sustainable weight loss, improved mental focus, and increased energy levels.

But "The Keto Code" goes beyond just the basics.

We will explore the science behind ketosis, diving into the mechanisms that make this dietary approach so effective.

You'll learn about the role of insulin, the importance of macronutrient ratios, and how to optimize your nutrient intake to maximize your results.

Moreover, this book will serve as your culinary companion, featuring a collection of mouthwatering recipes specifically designed for the ketogenic diet.

From breakfast staples to savory main courses and decadent desserts, you'll discover that eating keto doesn't mean sacrificing flavor or variety.

Get ready to enjoy meals that nourish your body and delight your taste buds.

"The Keto Code" also addresses common challenges and provides practical strategies for overcoming them.

We'll tackle the dreaded keto flu, teach you how to navigate dining out while staying in ketosis, and offer tips for maintaining your progress during social events.

This is a lifestyle, not a temporary fix, and we're here to ensure you have all the tools you need to succeed.

So, are you ready to embark on a transformative journey? Prepare to unlock the secrets of weight loss and optimal health through the power of "The Keto Code."

Let's decode the mysteries together and embrace a lifestyle that will revolutionize the way you look, feel, and live. Get ready to take the first step towards a healthier, more vibrant you.

It's time to unlock the code.

Chapter 1

Introduction - Cracking the Code

Weight loss can often feel like an elusive puzzle, leaving many individuals frustrated and overwhelmed.

With countless diets and approaches vying for attention, it's challenging to discern which path will lead to lasting results.

In "The Keto Code: Unlocking the Secrets of Weight Loss and Optimal Health," we invite you to embark on a transformative journey that will unravel the mysteries and empower you to achieve your desired goals.

Understanding the Challenges of Weight Loss

To effectively address weight loss, it is crucial to understand the challenges associated with it.

Various factors contribute to weight management difficulties, including metabolic differences, hormonal imbalances, and genetic predispositions.

Traditional diets that rely on calorie restriction often fail to account for these complexities, leading to short-term success but long-term frustration.

Introducing the Ketogenic Lifestyle

The ketogenic diet, or keto for short, has emerged as a revolutionary approach to weight loss and overall health.

Unlike conventional diets that primarily focus on reducing fat intake, the ketogenic lifestyle centers around the concept of shifting the body's primary fuel source from carbohydrates to fat.

By significantly reducing carbohydrate consumption and increasing healthy fat intake, we can induce a state of ketosis.

Ketosis is a metabolic state in which the body turns to stored fats for energy, as opposed to relying on glucose derived from carbohydrates.

This metabolic shift has several profound effects on the body.

It not only leads to a significant reduction in body weight and body fat percentage but also offers other potential benefits such as improved insulin sensitivity, better blood sugar control, increased energy levels, and enhanced mental clarity.

Setting the Stage for Success

"The Keto Code" sets the stage for your success on the ketogenic journey.

By providing a comprehensive understanding of the principles behind the ketogenic lifestyle, you will be equipped with the knowledge needed to make informed decisions and achieve lasting results.

Throughout this book, we will delve into the science behind ketosis, exploring the mechanisms by which the body enters and sustains this metabolic state.

We will demystify the role of macronutrients—fats, proteins, and carbohydrates—and guide you in finding the optimal macronutrient ratios for your individual needs.

Understanding these ratios is essential in achieving and maintaining ketosis.

Creating a keto-friendly kitchen is crucial for your success.

In this chapter, we will help you stock your pantry with essential items that align with the principles of the ketogenic diet.

We will guide meal planning and grocery shopping, ensuring that you have the right ingredients to prepare delicious, satisfying meals that support your goals.

To kickstart your journey, we will guide you through the process of transitioning into a ketogenic lifestyle.

We will address common challenges and potential side effects, such as the "keto flu," and offer strategies to overcome them.

Additionally, we will provide tips for staying motivated, setting realistic expectations, and holding yourself accountable throughout the journey.

By cracking the code and understanding the intricacies of the ketogenic lifestyle, you will unlock the potential for sustained weight loss, improved health markers, and enhanced overall well-being.

"The Keto Code" is not a quick fix or a temporary solution.

It is a commitment to a lifestyle change that prioritizes your long-term health and vitality.

In the upcoming chapters, we will delve deeper into the science of ketosis, explore various meal options and recipes that align with the ketogenic principles, address common challenges you may encounter, and provide guidance on maintaining a healthy lifestyle beyond the initial phase.

Get ready to crack the code, embrace the power of the ketogenic lifestyle, and embark on a transformative journey that will revolutionize your relationship with food, reshape your body, and optimize your overall health.

Welcome to "The Keto Code: Unlocking the Secrets of Weight Loss and Optimal Health." Together, we will uncover the transformative potential of the ketogenic lifestyle and empower you to achieve the results you desire.

Chapter 2

Demystifying Ketosis

In this chapter, we will delve deeper into the science of ketosis, exploring how the body transitions into this state and the benefits it offers for weight loss and overall health.

By demystifying ketosis, you will gain a comprehensive understanding of the underlying mechanisms that make the ketogenic diet so effective.

The Science Behind Ketosis

Ketosis is a natural metabolic state in which the body utilizes stored fats as its primary source of fuel instead of carbohydrates.

To enter ketosis, it is necessary to restrict carbohydrate intake to a significant extent, typically below 50 grams per day.

This depletion of carbohydrates forces the body to seek alternative fuel sources, leading to the breakdown of stored fats into molecules called ketones.

Ketones serve as an efficient energy source for the body, particularly for the brain, which can readily utilize ketones for fuel.

When the concentration of ketones in the bloodstream reaches a certain level, the body is considered to be in a state of ketosis.

This metabolic shift has several profound effects on weight loss and overall health.

Benefits of Ketosis for Weight Loss

One of the primary reasons individuals turn to the ketogenic diet is its remarkable ability to promote weight loss.

When the body is in ketosis, it becomes highly efficient at burning stored fat for energy.

As a result, excess body fat is gradually reduced, leading to a reduction in overall body weight and body fat percentage.

Moreover, the ketogenic diet has been shown to help curb hunger and reduce cravings, making it easier to maintain a caloric deficit and adhere to a weight loss plan.

The steady supply of ketones also helps stabilize blood sugar levels, reducing fluctuations that can contribute to overeating and weight gain.

Beyond Weight Loss & Additional Health Benefits

While weight loss is a significant benefit of ketosis, the ketogenic lifestyle offers a range of additional health advantages.

Research has suggested that the ketogenic diet may improve insulin sensitivity, which is crucial for individuals with insulin resistance or type 2 diabetes.

By reducing carbohydrate intake, the ketogenic diet minimizes spikes in blood sugar levels, promoting better glycemic control. Ketosis has also been associated with improved cardiovascular health.

Studies have shown that the ketogenic diet can lead to a reduction in triglyceride levels, an increase in high-density lipoprotein (HDL) cholesterol (often referred to as "good" cholesterol), and a decrease in low-density lipoprotein (LDL) cholesterol (often referred to as "bad" cholesterol).

Furthermore, the ketogenic diet has shown promise in managing certain neurological conditions, such as epilepsy.

Ketones provide an alternative energy source for the brain, and their neuroprotective properties may help reduce seizures and improve cognitive function in individuals with epilepsy.

It is important to note that while the ketogenic lifestyle offers many potential benefits, it may not be suitable for everyone.

It is essential to consult with a healthcare professional before embarking on any dietary changes, especially if you have specific health concerns or conditions.

Understanding the Mechanisms of Ketosis

To fully grasp the mechanisms of ketosis, it is important to understand the role of insulin, a hormone secreted by the pancreas.

Insulin is primarily responsible for regulating blood sugar levels and facilitating the uptake of glucose into cells for energy.

When carbohydrate intake is high, the body releases insulin to help transport glucose from the bloodstream into cells.

This leads to an increase in blood sugar levels, as excess glucose is stored as glycogen in the liver and muscles.

However, when carbohydrate intake is reduced, insulin levels decrease, prompting the body to shift to alternative fuel sources.

As insulin levels decrease, the hormone glucagon is released, signaling the liver to break down stored glycogen into glucose.

This process, known as glycogenolysis, helps maintain stable blood sugar levels during the initial stages of carbohydrate restriction.

Once the liver's glycogen stores are depleted, the body turns to fat stores for fuel.

Fatty acids are released from adipose tissue and transported to the liver, where they undergo a process called beta-oxidation, breaking down fatty acids into molecules called ketones.

These ketones are then released into the bloodstream and serve as an energy source for various tissues, including the brain.

As the body adapts to utilizing ketones for fuel, the production and utilization of ketones become more efficient.

This transition typically takes several days to a few weeks, during which individuals may experience temporary side effects such as fatigue, headaches, and irritability.

This period, often referred to as the "keto flu," is a common occurrence as the body adjusts to the metabolic shift.

Understanding the science of ketosis is key to harnessing the power of the ketogenic lifestyle.

By entering a state of ketosis, the body becomes a fat-burning machine, promoting weight loss and offering a range of potential health benefits.

From improved insulin sensitivity and cardiovascular health to managing neurological conditions, the ketogenic diet has demonstrated its efficacy.

In the upcoming chapters, we will explore how to find the optimal macronutrient ratios for ketosis, provide guidance on creating keto-friendly meals, and address common challenges and misconceptions associated with the ketogenic lifestyle.

By mastering the principles of ketosis, you will be empowered to unlock the full potential of the ketogenic code and achieve your weight loss and health goals.

Chapter 3

The Power of Macronutrients

Now, in this Chapter, we will delve into the role of macronutrients—fats, proteins, and carbohydrates—in the ketogenic diet.

Understanding the power of macronutrients is essential for finding the optimal balance that supports ketosis and promotes weight loss and overall health.

Understanding Fats, Proteins, and Carbohydrates

Macronutrients are the three main categories of nutrients that provide energy to the body.

Each macronutrient plays a distinct role in metabolism and has unique characteristics that influence our health and well-being.

1-Fats

Fats are a critical component of the ketogenic diet as they serve as the primary source of energy when the body is in ketosis.

They provide a concentrated source of energy and play crucial roles in hormone production, insulation of vital organs, and absorption of fat-soluble vitamins.

It is important to focus on consuming healthy fats, such as monounsaturated fats (found in olive oil, avocados, and nuts) and polyunsaturated fats (found in fatty fish, flaxseeds, and walnuts).

These fats provide essential fatty acids, such as omega-3 and omega-6, which have been associated with numerous health benefits, including reduced inflammation and improved heart health.

2-Proteins

Proteins are the building blocks of the body, essential for the growth, repair, and maintenance of tissues, enzymes, and hormones.

While the ketogenic diet is often characterized as high in fat, it also includes an adequate intake of protein.

When it comes to protein consumption on a ketogenic diet, it is important to focus on quality sources such as lean meats, poultry, fish, eggs, and plant-based protein sources like tofu, tempeh, and legumes.

These protein sources not only provide essential amino acids but also offer additional nutrients and minerals necessary for optimal health.

3-Carbohydrates

Carbohydrates are the macronutrient that has the greatest impact on blood sugar levels.

In the ketogenic diet, carbohydrate intake is significantly restricted to induce and maintain ketosis.

By minimizing carbohydrate consumption, we reduce the body's reliance on glucose as its primary fuel source.

When following a ketogenic diet, it is crucial to choose carbohydrates wisely.

Most carbohydrates should come from nutrient-dense sources such as non-starchy vegetables, leafy greens, and small amounts of low-glycemic fruits.

These carbohydrates provide essential fiber, vitamins, and minerals while minimizing the impact on blood sugar levels.

Finding the Optimal Macronutrient Ratio for Ketosis

The key to achieving and maintaining ketosis lies in finding the optimal macronutrient ratio for your individual needs.

While there is no one-size-fits-all approach, a common guideline for a standard ketogenic diet (SKD) is to consume approximately 70-75% of daily calories from fat, 20-25% from protein, and 5-10% from carbohydrates.

It is important to note that these percentages are general recommendations, and individual needs may vary.

Factors such as activity level, metabolic rate, and specific health conditions should be considered when determining the appropriate macronutrient ratio.

Consulting with a healthcare professional or registered dietitian can provide personalized guidance based on your unique circumstances.

Calculating and Tracking Macros for Success

To effectively follow a ketogenic diet, it is helpful to calculate and track your macronutrient intake.

Various online tools and mobile apps are available to assist in this process.

By tracking your macros, you can ensure that you are staying within your desired macronutrient ranges and maximizing your chances of achieving and maintaining ketosis.

It is important to maintain a balance of macronutrients and not solely focus on one category.

Consuming excessive protein or carbohydrates may hinder ketosis and impede weight loss progress.

By monitoring your macros, you can make necessary adjustments and optimize your dietary intake for success.

Understanding the power of macronutrients is crucial for effectively following the ketogenic diet.

By finding the optimal balance of fats, proteins, and carbohydrates, you can support ketosis, promote weight loss, and enhance overall health.

Focus on consuming healthy fats, quality proteins, and nutrient-dense carbohydrates while tracking your macros to ensure you are on the right path toward achieving your desired goals.

In the next chapter, we will explore practical strategies for creating delicious and satisfying meals that align with the principles of the ketogenic lifestyle.

Chapter 4

Crafting Delicious and Nutritious Keto Meals

Now, in this Chapter, we will explore practical strategies for crafting delicious and nutritious meals that align with the principles of the ketogenic lifestyle.

By focusing on flavorful ingredients and creative combinations, you can enjoy a variety of satisfying dishes while maintaining ketosis and promoting optimal health.

Building a Keto-Friendly Pantry

A well-stocked pantry is the foundation of successful meal preparation on the ketogenic diet.

By having the right ingredients on hand, you can easily create flavorful and satisfying meals that support your goals.

Here are some essential items to include in your keto-friendly pantry:

1. **Healthy Fats**

Olive oil, coconut oil, avocados, nuts (such as almonds, walnuts, and macadamia nuts), and seeds (such as chia seeds, flaxseeds, and hemp seeds) are excellent sources of healthy fats.

These ingredients provide richness and flavor to your dishes while keeping you satiated.

2. **Protein Sources**

Choose a variety of high-quality protein sources, including lean meats (such as chicken, turkey, and grass-fed beef), fatty fish (like salmon and sardines), eggs, and plant-based protein options (such as tofu, tempeh, and seitan).

3. **Low-Carb Vegetables**

Non-starchy vegetables are a vital component of the ketogenic diet as they provide fiber, essential vitamins, and minerals while being low in carbohydrates.

Stock up on leafy greens (such as spinach, kale, and arugula), cruciferous vegetables (like broccoli, cauliflower, and Brussels sprouts), as well as zucchini, bell peppers, and mushrooms.

4. Flavorful Herbs and Spices

Enhance the taste of your meals with an assortment of herbs and spices.

Common options include basil, oregano, thyme, rosemary, cumin, turmeric, paprika, garlic powder, and onion powder.

Creating Balanced and Flavorful Keto Meals

Crafting delicious and nutritious keto meals requires a careful balance of macronutrients while prioritizing flavor and variety. Here are some strategies to consider:

1. **Focus on Healthy Fats**:

Make healthy fats the star of your meals by incorporating ingredients like avocado, olive oil, coconut oil, and nuts , These fats add richness and depth of flavor while providing satiety.

2. Adequate Protein

Ensure each meal includes a sufficient amount of protein to support muscle maintenance and promote satiety.

Opt for lean meats, fatty fish, eggs, or plant-based protein sources.

3. Embrace Non-Starchy Vegetables

Fill your plate with a variety of non-starchy vegetables to add color, texture, and valuable nutrients to your meals.

Consider roasting or sautéing them with herbs and spices for added flavor.

4. Experiment with Herbs and Spices

Elevate the taste of your dishes by incorporating a diverse range of herbs and spices.

Experiment with different combinations to discover unique flavor profiles that keep your meals exciting and enjoyable.

5. Be Mindful of Carbohydrate Content

Keep an eye on the carbohydrate content of ingredients you use, especially when incorporating fruits, nuts, and dairy products.

While these items can be part of a ketogenic diet, moderation is key to staying within your desired macronutrient ranges.

Meal Planning and Preparation

Meal planning and preparation are essential for staying on track with your ketogenic lifestyle.

By dedicating time to plan your meals and prepare them in advance, you can save time, reduce stress, and ensure that you always have keto-friendly options readily available, Here are some tips:

1. Plan your meals for the week, taking into consideration your macronutrient goals and personal preferences.

2. Create a grocery list based on your meal plan and stock up on fresh ingredients.

3. Dedicate a specific time each week for meal preparation. Cook and portion out meals in advance, so they are easily accessible throughout the week.

4. Consider batch cooking staple items like proteins, roasted vegetables, and sauces that can be used in multiple meals.

5. Explore meal prepping techniques such as freezer-friendly recipes or utilizing slow cookers and Instant Pots for convenient and time-saving options.

Crafting delicious and nutritious keto meals is an essential aspect of maintaining the ketogenic lifestyle.

By building a keto-friendly pantry, focusing on healthy fats, incorporating adequate protein, embracing non-starchy vegetables, and exploring a variety of herbs and spices, you can create flavorful and satisfying dishes that support your goals.

Additionally, meal planning and preparation are valuable tools for staying consistent and ensuring you have convenient and wholesome options available.

In the next chapter, we will address common challenges faced on the ketogenic journey and provide strategies to overcome them, helping you stay motivated and committed to your path of success.

Chapter 5

Overcoming Challenges on the Ketogenic Journey

Now, in this Chapter, we will address the common challenges faced on the ketogenic journey and provide strategies to overcome them.

By understanding and proactively addressing these challenges, you can stay motivated, committed, and successful in achieving your health and weight loss goals.

1-Dealing with Keto Flu:

During the initial stages of transitioning into ketosis, some individuals may experience what is known as the "keto flu." Symptoms can include fatigue, headaches, irritability, and brain fog.

While these symptoms are temporary and typically resolve within a few days to a week, they can be challenging to manage. Here are some strategies to alleviate the keto flu:

. Stay Hydrated:

Drink plenty of water and replenish electrolytes, as the body excretes more water and minerals during the early stages of ketosis. Consider incorporating electrolyte-rich beverages or supplementing with electrolyte powders.

. Increase Salt Intake:

As carbohydrate intake decreases, insulin levels drop, leading to increased excretion of sodium. Adding a bit more salt to your meals or consuming broth can help maintain proper electrolyte balance.

. Gradual Carbohydrate Reduction:

Gradually reducing carbohydrate intake over a week or two instead of making drastic changes can help ease the transition into ketosis and minimize keto flu symptoms.

2-Dining Out and Social Events

Navigating social situations and dining out while following a ketogenic diet can present challenges.

However, with a little planning and flexibility, you can enjoy social gatherings while staying true to your dietary goals. Here are some strategies:

. Research Menu Options:

Check the menu of the restaurant you'll be visiting in advance and look for keto-friendly options.

Many establishments now offer low-carb or customizable choices.

. Focus on Protein and Vegetables:

Opt for protein-rich dishes such as grilled chicken or fish and pair them with non-starchy vegetables.

Request modifications, such as substituting high-carb sides with additional vegetables.

. Be Prepared with Keto Snacks:

Carry keto-friendly snacks like nuts, seeds, or jerky in your bag or car to help curb cravings and avoid giving in to temptations.

. Communicate Your Dietary Needs:

Inform your friends, family, or hosts about your dietary preferences beforehand, so they can accommodate your needs or offer alternatives.

3-Plateau and Lack of Progress

Experiencing a plateau or a lack of progress can be disheartening, especially after initial success.

However, it's important to remember that weight loss journeys have ups and downs.

Here are strategies to overcome plateaus and maintain progress:

. Revisit Macros and Caloric Intake:

Double-check your macronutrient ratios and caloric intake to ensure they align with your current needs. Adjustments may be necessary as your body adapts and your weight changes.

. Increase Physical Activity:

Incorporate regular exercise or switch up your workout routine to challenge your body and boost your metabolism. Strength training can be particularly beneficial for building lean muscle mass.

. Practice Intermittent Fasting:

Intermittent fasting, which involves alternating periods of fasting and eating, can help break through plateaus and enhance fat-burning.

Consult with a healthcare professional before starting any fasting regimen.

. Manage Stress and Sleep:

Chronic stress and inadequate sleep can impact weight loss progress.

Prioritize self-care, engage in stress-reducing activities, and ensure you get quality sleep to support your body's natural processes.

4-Staying Motivated and Focused

Maintaining motivation throughout your ketogenic journey is crucial for long-term success.

Here are strategies to stay motivated and focused:

. Set Realistic Goals:

Set realistic, attainable goals that align with your overall health objectives.

Break them down into smaller milestones, celebrating each achievement along the way.

. Track Progress:

Keep a food and mood journal to track your meals, macros, and emotions.

This can provide valuable insights into patterns and help identify areas for improvement.

. Seek Support and Accountability:

Join online communities, participate in support groups, or find an accountability partner who shares your goals.

Sharing experiences, exchanging tips, and having someone to lean on can boost motivation and encourage.

. Celebrate Non-Scale Victories:

Shift the focus from solely relying on the scale.

Celebrate non-scale victories such as improved energy levels, clothing fit, increased strength, or enhanced mental clarity.

. Embrace Variety and Flexibility:

Explore new recipes, experiment with different ingredients, and embrace the flexibility of the ketogenic lifestyle.

This can prevent monotony, keep meals exciting, and prevent feelings of deprivation.

In this Chapter, has addressed common challenges encountered on the ketogenic journey and provided strategies to overcome them.

 By acknowledging the possibility of the keto flu, planning for social situations, navigating plateaus, and staying motivated, you can overcome obstacles and continue making progress toward your health and weight loss goals.

Remember, the ketogenic lifestyle is a long-term commitment, and with perseverance and the right strategies, you can achieve sustainable success.

In the next chapter, we will explore additional tips and tricks to optimize your ketogenic experience and maintain a healthy, balanced lifestyle.

Chapter 6

Optimizing Your Ketogenic Lifestyle

Now, in this Chapter, we will explore additional tips and tricks to optimize your ketogenic lifestyle.

By implementing these strategies, you can enhance the effectiveness of the ketogenic diet, promote overall well-being, and maintain a healthy, balanced lifestyle.

1-Prioritizing Nutrient Density

While achieving and maintaining ketosis is essential, it's equally important to focus on the nutrient density of your food choices.

Opt for whole, unprocessed foods that provide a wide range of vitamins, minerals, and antioxidants.

Prioritize nutrient-dense options such as leafy greens, colorful vegetables, berries, fatty fish, and quality sources of protein.

This approach ensures that your body receives the essential nutrients it needs for optimal health.

2-Practicing Mindful Eating

Mindful eating involves paying attention to your body's hunger and fullness cues, as well as savoring and enjoying each bite.

By slowing down, chewing your food thoroughly, and being present during meals, you can enhance digestion, improve satisfaction, and prevent overeating.

Mindful eating also allows you to develop a deeper connection with your body, promoting a positive relationship with food.

3-Incorporating Intermittent Fasting

Intermittent fasting is an eating pattern that involves cycling between periods of fasting and eating.

It can complement the ketogenic diet by enhancing fat-burning and promoting metabolic flexibility.

Consider incorporating intermittent fasting protocols such as the 16:8 method (fasting for 16 hours, followed by an 8-hour eating window) or the 24-hour fast once or twice a week.

However, it's important to consult with a healthcare professional before starting any fasting regimen, especially if you have underlying health conditions.

4-Managing Stress and Sleep

Chronic stress and inadequate sleep can impact your overall health and hinder weight loss progress. Incorporate stress management techniques such as meditation, deep breathing exercises, yoga, or engaging in hobbies that bring you joy.

Additionally, prioritize quality sleep by establishing a consistent bedtime routine, creating a relaxing sleep environment, and ensuring you get the recommended 7-9 hours of sleep per night.

Proper stress management and sufficient sleep support hormonal balance, metabolism, and overall well-being.

5-Incorporating Physical Activity

Regular physical activity is beneficial for both physical and mental health.

Engage in activities that you enjoy, such as walking, jogging, cycling, swimming, or strength training. Exercise can enhance fat burning, improve cardiovascular health, boost mood, and increase overall energy levels.

Aim for a combination of cardiovascular exercises and strength training to promote muscle growth and maintenance.

6-Practicing Self-Care and Mindset

Taking care of your mental and emotional well-being is essential on the ketogenic journey.

Practice self-care activities that promote relaxation and stress reduction, such as taking baths, reading, journaling, or spending time in nature.

Cultivate a positive mindset by focusing on self-compassion, gratitude, and celebrating progress. Surround yourself with a supportive network of friends and family who uplift and encourage you on your journey.

7-Regular Monitoring and Adjustments

Monitoring your progress and making necessary adjustments is crucial for long-term success.

Regularly assess your body composition, energy levels, and overall well-being.

Consider tracking key metrics such as weight, body measurements, and blood markers to gauge progress. Based on these measurements and feedback from your body, make appropriate adjustments to your macronutrient ratios, caloric intake, or exercise routine to continue optimizing your ketogenic lifestyle.

This Chapter has provided additional tips and strategies to optimize your ketogenic lifestyle.

By prioritizing nutrient density, practicing mindful eating, incorporating intermittent fasting, managing stress and sleep, engaging in physical activity, practicing self-care and cultivating a positive mindset, and regularly monitoring and adjusting your approach, you can enhance the effectiveness of the ketogenic diet and maintain a balanced, healthy lifestyle.

Remember, the ketogenic journey is unique to each individual, so it's essential to listen to your body's needs and make personalized adjustments along the way.

In the final chapter, we will summarize the key takeaways and provide a roadmap for long-term success on the ketogenic journey.

Chapter 7:

Sustaining Long-Term Success on the Ketogenic Journey

We will summarize the key takeaways and provide a roadmap for sustaining long-term success on the ketogenic journey.

By incorporating these principles into your daily life, you can maintain the benefits of the ketogenic diet while enjoying improved health, sustainable weight management, and overall well-being.

1-Embrace a Lifestyle, Not a Diet

The ketogenic approach is more than just a temporary diet; it is a lifestyle change.

Embrace the mindset that prioritizes nourishing your body with wholesome, nutrient-dense foods and making sustainable choices.

Instead of viewing it as a short-term fix, shift your focus to long-term health and well-being.

2- Find Your Sustainable Macronutrient Balance

While there are general guidelines for macronutrient ratios on a ketogenic diet, it's essential to find the balance that works best for your body and goals.

Pay attention to how different macronutrient ratios make you feel, monitor your progress, and adjust accordingly. Experiment with variations in fat, protein, and carbohydrate intake to find what helps you achieve and maintain ketosis while supporting your individual needs.

3- Focus on Whole, Unprocessed Foods

To optimize your ketogenic lifestyle, prioritize whole, unprocessed foods.

These include lean proteins, healthy fats, non-starchy vegetables, nuts, seeds, and berries.

Minimize consumption of processed foods, refined grains, added sugars, and artificial ingredients.

By choosing nutrient-dense options, you provide your body with essential vitamins, minerals, and antioxidants for optimal health.

4-Practice Mindful Eating and Portion Control

Continuing to practice mindful eating and portion control is crucial for long-term success.

Pay attention to your body's hunger and fullness cues, savor each bite, and eat until you feel satisfied rather than stuffed.

Be mindful of portion sizes to ensure you maintain an appropriate caloric intake for your goals.

4. Keep Learning and Experimenting

The world of nutrition and health is constantly evolving.

Stay informed by keeping up with the latest research, seeking out credible sources of information, and learning from experts in the field.

Remain open to new ideas and be willing to experiment with different approaches to optimize your ketogenic journey.

6-Foster a Supportive Environment

Surround yourself with a supportive environment that encourages and uplifts you on your ketogenic journey. Seek out like-minded individuals, whether through online communities, support groups, or local meetups.

Share your experiences, exchange tips, and provide support to others.

Having a support system can greatly enhance your motivation, accountability, and overall success.

7-Practice Flexibility and Balance

While the ketogenic lifestyle has clear guidelines, it's important to maintain flexibility and balance.

Allow yourself occasional indulgences or deviations from the strictest interpretation of the diet.

Social occasions, special events, and personal preferences may call for some modifications or temporary adjustments.

Remember, sustainable success is built on finding a balance that works for you while still adhering to the core principles of the ketogenic approach.

8. Regular Evaluation and Reflection

Periodically evaluate and reflect on your progress, goals, and overall well-being.

Assess how the ketogenic lifestyle is positively impacting various aspects of your life, including your energy levels, mood, body composition, and overall health markers. Celebrate achievements, reassess goals, and make any necessary adjustments to maintain your momentum and continue progressing on your journey.

This Chapter has outlined the key principles for sustaining long-term success on the ketogenic journey. By embracing it as a lifestyle, finding your sustainable macronutrient balance, focusing on whole, unprocessed foods, practicing mindful eating, staying open to learning, fostering a supportive environment, practicing flexibility and balance, and regularly evaluating and reflecting on your progress, you can maintain the benefits of the ketogenic lifestyle for years to come.

Remember, this is a personal journey, and each individual's path will be unique.

Stay committed, stay curious, and enjoy the many rewards that come with living a healthy and fulfilling ketogenic lifestyle.

Chapter 8

Beyond the Ketogenic Lifestyle

In the previous chapters, we have explored the ins and outs of the ketogenic lifestyle, from understanding the science behind ketosis to implementing strategies for long-term success.

Now, in Chapter, we will delve into the realm of expanding your horizons beyond the ketogenic diet. While the ketogenic approach can offer numerous health benefits, it's important to explore other aspects of wellness that can complement and enhance your overall well-being.

1-Mind-Body Connection:

The mind-body connection plays a vital role in our overall health and wellness.

Consider incorporating practices that promote mental and emotional well-being alongside your ketogenic journey.

This may include mindfulness meditation, yoga, deep breathing exercises, journaling, or engaging in activities that bring you joy and reduce stress.

Cultivating a positive mindset and nurturing your mental and emotional health can have profound effects on your overall well-being.

2-Exercise and Movement:

Physical activity goes hand in hand with a healthy lifestyle.

While the ketogenic diet can provide energy and support weight management, regular exercise and movement are crucial for cardiovascular health, strength, flexibility, and overall fitness.

Explore different forms of exercise that you enjoy, such as strength training, cardio workouts, yoga, or outdoor activities.

Find a balance between resistance training to build lean muscle mass and cardiovascular exercises to improve heart health.

3-Sleep Optimization:

Quality sleep is often overlooked but is crucial for optimal health.

Prioritize creating a sleep-friendly environment, establishing a consistent bedtime routine, and getting the recommended 7-9 hours of sleep per night.

Avoid stimulating activities before bed, limit exposure to screens, and create a relaxing atmosphere in your bedroom.

Quality sleep supports hormone regulation, cognitive function, immune health, and overall vitality.

4-Stress Management:

Chronic stress can take a toll on both our physical and mental well-being. Explore various stress management techniques to find what works best for you.

This may include practices such as meditation, deep breathing exercises, nature walks, engaging in hobbies, or seeking support from a therapist or counselor.

By managing stress effectively, you can improve your overall resilience and maintain a balanced, healthy lifestyle.

5-Building Healthy Relationships:

Nurturing healthy relationships is an essential aspect of overall well-being.

Surround yourself with supportive individuals who uplift and encourage you on your journey.

Foster open communication, practice empathy, and establish boundaries to maintain healthy connections.

Building meaningful relationships can provide a sense of belonging, support, and fulfillment in your life.

6-Lifelong Learning:

Continued education and learning can be incredibly enriching.

Expand your knowledge beyond nutrition and explore other areas of interest that align with your passions.

This may include exploring new hobbies, taking up a creative pursuit, enrolling in courses or workshops, or diving into personal development books.

Lifelong learning keeps the mind engaged, promotes personal growth, and can add depth and richness to your life.

7-Regular Health Check-ups:

While the ketogenic lifestyle can have significant health benefits, it's important to prioritize regular health check-ups and screenings.

Schedule routine visits with your healthcare provider to monitor your overall health, assess any potential nutrient deficiencies, and discuss any concerns or questions you may have.

Regular check-ups ensure that you stay proactive in maintaining your well-being.

8-Environmental Considerations:

The environment we live in can significantly impact our health and well-being.

Consider exploring ways to make your living environment more conducive to a healthy lifestyle.

This may include creating a clutter-free and organized space, incorporating plants for improved air quality, using natural cleaning products, reducing exposure to toxins, and spending time in nature.

Taking steps to create an environmentally friendly and sustainable living environment can contribute to your overall wellness.

9-Emotional Well-being:

Emotional well-being is an essential aspect of leading a fulfilling life.

Explore techniques and practices that promote emotional balance and resilience.

This may include seeking therapy or counseling to address past traumas or emotional challenges, practicing self-compassion, engaging in activities that bring you joy, and expressing your emotions in healthy ways. Cultivating emotional well-being allows you to navigate life's ups and downs with greater ease and contentment.

10-Purpose and Meaning:

Finding purpose and meaning in your life can provide a sense of fulfillment and direction.

Reflect on your values, passions, and interests to discover what brings meaning to your life.

This may involve pursuing a career that aligns with your values, volunteering for causes you believe in, or engaging in activities that contribute to the well-being of others.

Connecting with a sense of purpose can bring a profound sense of fulfillment and satisfaction to your journey.

11-Personal Growth and Resilience:

Personal growth involves continuous self-improvement and development.

Explore practices that promote personal growth and enhance your resilience.

This may include setting goals, challenging yourself to step outside your comfort zone, seeking opportunities for learning and growth, and embracing failure as a learning experience.

By fostering personal growth and building resilience, you can navigate life's challenges with greater strength and adaptability.

12-Cultivating Gratitude:

Practicing gratitude involves intentionally focusing on the positive aspects of your life and expressing gratitude for them. E

xplore ways to cultivate gratitude in your daily life, such as keeping a gratitude journal, expressing appreciation to others, or engaging in gratitude meditations.

Cultivating gratitude can shift your perspective, enhance your overall well-being, and foster a greater sense of contentment and happiness.

13-Giving Back and Service:

Contributing to the well-being of others through acts of kindness and service can bring immense fulfillment and purpose to your life.

Explore opportunities to give back to your community or support causes that resonate with you.

This may involve volunteering your time, donating to charitable organizations, or participating in community service projects.

Giving back not only benefits others but also enhances your sense of purpose and connection with the world around you.

14-Adapting and Evolving:

Remember that wellness is a dynamic and ever-evolving journey.

Be open to adapting and refining your approach as you gain new insights and experiences.

Continuously reassess your goals, values, and priorities to ensure they align with your evolving needs.

Embrace flexibility and embrace the opportunity for growth and positive change along your path.

This Chapter has emphasized the importance of expanding your horizons beyond the ketogenic lifestyle to encompass various aspects of wellness.

By considering the mind-body connection, incorporating exercise, optimizing sleep, managing stress, building healthy relationships, embracing lifelong learning, considering environmental factors, nurturing emotional well-being, finding purpose and meaning, promoting personal growth, cultivating gratitude, giving back, and remaining adaptable, you can create a holistic approach to your well-being.

Remember, wellness is a lifelong journey, and by exploring these additional dimensions, you can experience a more fulfilling and vibrant life.

Chapter 9

Navigating Challenges and Maintaining Motivation

In the previous chapters, we have explored the various aspects of the ketogenic lifestyle, from understanding its principles to expanding our horizons beyond diet and nutrition.

Now, in this Chapter, we will address the common challenges that arise on the ketogenic journey and provide strategies for navigating them effectively. Additionally, we will discuss how to maintain motivation and stay committed to your health and wellness goals in the face of obstacles.

1-Overcoming Plateaus:

Plateaus are a common occurrence on any wellness journey, including the ketogenic lifestyle.

When weight loss or other desired outcomes stall, it's important not to get discouraged.

Instead, consider making adjustments to your macronutrient ratios, tracking your food intake more diligently, or incorporating intermittent fasting to break through the plateau.

Stay patient and trust the process, as plateaus are often temporary.

2-Dealing with Social Pressures:

Navigating social situations and managing the pressures of external influences can be challenging on the ketogenic journey.

Friends and family may not fully understand or support your dietary choices, leading to feelings of isolation or temptation to deviate from your plan.

Communicate your goals and reasons for following a ketogenic lifestyle, and seek support from like-minded individuals.

Plan for social gatherings by bringing your keto-friendly options or suggesting restaurants with suitable choices.

Remember that your health and well-being are a priority, and stay true to your intentions.

3-Traveling and Dining Out:

Maintaining a ketogenic lifestyle while traveling or dining out requires some planning and flexibility.

Research restaurants in advance to identify keto-friendly options and familiarize yourself with local cuisine.

Pack keto-friendly snacks for travel and be prepared to make adjustments or substitutions to fit your dietary needs.

Focus on protein and vegetable-based meals, and communicate your dietary requirements to the waitstaff. With a little preparation, you can enjoy your travel experiences while staying on track with your ketogenic goals.

4-Dealing with Cravings and Emotional Eating:
Cravings and emotional eating can pose challenges on the ketogenic journey.

It's important to distinguish between true hunger and emotional triggers.

Practice mindful eating and self-awareness to identify the underlying causes of cravings.

Find alternative strategies to cope with emotions, such as engaging in physical activity, practicing relaxation techniques, or reaching out to a support system.

Incorporating satisfying keto-friendly treats or finding creative ways to recreate your favorite comfort foods can also help manage cravings more healthily.

5-Managing Keto Flu and Side Effects:

During the initial transition to ketosis, some individuals may experience "keto flu" symptoms such as fatigue, headaches, or irritability.

These side effects are typically temporary and can be managed by staying well-hydrated, replenishing electrolytes, and ensuring adequate rest.

Incorporating nutrient-dense foods and exploring supplements like magnesium or exogenous ketones may also provide relief.

Remember that your body is adapting to a new metabolic state, and with time, these side effects should subside.

6-Staying Motivated:

Maintaining motivation is crucial for long-term success on the ketogenic journey.

Set clear and realistic goals, both short-term and long-term, and regularly revisit and revise them as needed. Celebrate your achievements along the way, no matter how small, to stay motivated.

Surround yourself with positive influences, whether it be through supportive communities, motivational podcasts, or inspiring literature.

Additionally, find activities or hobbies that bring you joy and make you feel accomplished, reinforcing your commitment to overall well-being.

7-Seeking Professional Guidance:

If you find yourself facing persistent challenges or feel overwhelmed, seeking professional guidance from a registered dietitian or healthcare provider experienced in ketogenic nutrition can be beneficial.

They can provide personalized guidance, address specific concerns, and offer valuable insights to help you navigate the complexities of the ketogenic lifestyle.

Remember that you don't have to go through this journey alone, and seeking support from experts can enhance your success.

8-Balancing Macros and Micros:

Achieving the right balance of macronutrients (fat, protein, and carbohydrates) is crucial for success on the ketogenic diet.

However, it's equally important to pay attention to micronutrients (vitamins and minerals) to ensure optimal health and well-being.

Include a variety of nutrient-dense foods in your diet, such as leafy greens, cruciferous vegetables, nuts, seeds, and high-quality sources of protein.

Consider tracking your food intake using a reliable app or working with a registered dietitian to ensure you're meeting your nutritional needs.

9-Dealing with Setbacks:

Setbacks are a natural part of any journey, and the ketogenic lifestyle is no exception.

Whether it's a temporary lapse in adherence or a significant deviation from your plan, it's important to approach setbacks with compassion and a growth mindset.

Learn from the experience, identify triggers or underlying factors that led to the setback, and recommit to your goals.

Don't let setbacks discourage you; view them as opportunities for learning and growth.

10-Addressing Food Sensitivities:

Food sensitivities can sometimes interfere with your progress on the ketogenic journey.

If you suspect you have sensitivities to certain foods, consider implementing an elimination diet or working with a healthcare professional to identify trigger foods. While the ketogenic diet itself can often reduce inflammation and alleviate symptoms related to food sensitivities, it's important to address any underlying issues to optimize your health and well-being.

11-Finding Support and Accountability:

Having a support system and accountability partners can significantly enhance your success on the ketogenic journey.

Join online communities, participate in support groups, or find an accountability buddy who shares similar goals.

Connecting with others who understand the challenges and triumphs of the ketogenic lifestyle can provide motivation, inspiration, and a sense of belonging.

Share your experiences, ask for advice, and offer support to others in return.

12-Practicing Self-Care:

Self-care is a vital component of maintaining motivation and well-being on the ketogenic journey.

Take time to prioritize self-care activities that nourish your body, mind, and soul.

This may include engaging in relaxation techniques, taking baths, practicing mindfulness or meditation, engaging in hobbies, or simply spending time in nature. Recognize that self-care is not selfish but necessary for recharging and rejuvenating yourself along the way.

13-Periodic Reevaluation:

As you progress on your ketogenic journey, periodically reassess and reevaluate your goals and strategies.

Our bodies and lifestyles can change over time, and it's important to adapt your approach accordingly.

Reflect on your progress, assess what's working well, and identify areas for improvement.

This process of reflection and adjustment ensures that you stay aligned with your evolving needs and continue to make progress toward your health and wellness goals.

14-Embracing Long-Term Lifestyle Changes:

Ultimately, the ketogenic lifestyle is not just a temporary diet but a long-term commitment to health and well-being.

Embrace the idea of sustainable lifestyle changes rather than viewing it as a short-term fix.

Gradually integrate the principles of the ketogenic lifestyle into your daily routine, making it a seamless and enjoyable part of your life.

Emphasize whole, nutrient-dense foods, listen to your body's signals, and cultivate a positive relationship with food and your overall well-being.

This Chapter has explored the various challenges that can arise on the ketogenic journey and provided strategies for navigating them effectively.

By balancing macros and micros, addressing setbacks and food sensitivities, seeking support, practicing self-care, periodically reevaluating your approach, and embracing long-term lifestyle changes, you can overcome obstacles and maintain your motivation on this transformative journey.

Chapter 10

Sustaining Long-Term Success Introduction:

In this final chapter, we will delve into the key strategies and principles for sustaining long-term success on your ketogenic journey.

While the initial stages may have focused on adopting the ketogenic lifestyle, this chapter will guide you on how to maintain your progress, make the necessary adjustments, and embrace a sustainable approach to health and wellness.

1-Mindful Eating and Intuitive Awareness:

Mindful eating involves cultivating a heightened awareness of your body's hunger and fullness cues, as well as the sensory experience of eating.

Practice slowing down during meals, savoring each bite, and tuning into your body's signals of satiety.

By fostering a deeper connection with your body's needs and preferences, you can make informed choices that align with your health goals and prevent overeating or emotional eating.

2-Regular Physical Activity:

Physical activity is a vital component of overall health and plays a significant role in sustaining long-term success on the ketogenic journey.

Find forms of exercise that you enjoy and make them a regular part of your routine.

This can include activities such as strength training, cardiovascular exercises, yoga, or any other form of movement that brings you joy.

Regular physical activity not only supports weight management but also promotes cardiovascular health, improves mood, and enhances overall well-being.

3-Mindset and Self-Reflection:

Cultivating a positive mindset and engaging in self-reflection is key to sustaining long-term success.

Adopt a growth mindset, viewing challenges as opportunities for learning and growth rather than obstacles.

Regularly reflect on your progress, celebrate your achievements, and acknowledge areas for improvement. Engage in positive self-talk and practice self-compassion, fostering a nurturing inner dialogue that supports your ongoing journey toward optimal health and wellness.

4-Finding Balance and Flexibility:

Sustaining long-term success on the ketogenic journey requires finding a balance that works for you.

Embrace flexibility in your approach, allowing for occasional deviations or modifications to suit your lifestyle and preferences.

Remember that the ketogenic lifestyle is not a rigid set of rules but a framework that can be adapted to individual needs.

Find a balance that allows for the enjoyment of social occasions, special treats, and the occasional indulgence while still staying committed to your health goals.

5-Continued Learning and Growth:

Commit to lifelong learning and staying informed about the latest research and developments in the field of nutrition and wellness.

Stay curious and explore new recipes, techniques, and resources that can enhance your ketogenic journey. Consider attending workshops, seminars, or conferences related to nutrition and wellness to deepen your knowledge and expand your skill set.

By embracing a growth mindset and remaining open to new information, you can continuously refine your approach and stay motivated on your journey.

6-Tracking and Monitoring:

Maintaining awareness of your progress and outcomes is crucial for sustaining long-term success.

Consider tracking your food intake, macronutrient ratios, and key health markers to assess your progress and identify areas for improvement.

Utilize tools such as food diaries, mobile apps, or wearable devices to monitor your daily activities, sleep patterns, and other relevant metrics.

Regular tracking and monitoring provide valuable insights, accountability, and motivation to help you stay on track.

7-Cultivating a Supportive Environment:

Surround yourself with a supportive environment that aligns with your health goals.

Seek out like-minded individuals who share your interests in the ketogenic lifestyle or join supportive communities either online or offline.

Engage in positive social interactions, share your challenges and successes, and offer support to others in return.

By cultivating a supportive environment, you create a sense of camaraderie and accountability that can fuel your long-term success.

8-Celebrating Non-Scale Victories:

Shift your focus from solely relying on the scale as a measure of success.

Celebrate non-scale victories that go beyond weight loss, such as increased energy, improved mental clarity, enhanced physical performance, better sleep, or improved markers of overall health.

Acknowledge and celebrate these achievements as they demonstrate the positive impact of the ketogenic lifestyle on your well-being.

Recognizing and appreciating these non-scale victories will reinforce your commitment to long-term success.

9-Practicing Self-Care and Stress Management:

Self-care and stress management are essential for sustaining long-term success on the ketogenic journey.

Prioritize activities that promote relaxation and stress reduction, such as meditation, deep breathing exercises, spending time in nature, or engaging in hobbies and activities that bring you joy.

Recognize the importance of rest and recovery, ensuring you get adequate sleep each night.

By taking care of your mental and emotional well-being, you create a solid foundation for maintaining your health goals.

10-Setting Realistic Expectations:

Maintaining realistic expectations is crucial for sustaining long-term success.

Understand that progress may not always be linear, and there may be periods of plateaus or temporary setbacks. Avoid comparing your journey to others and focus on your progress and improvements.

Remember that lasting change takes time, and by setting realistic expectations, you can maintain a positive outlook and stay motivated for the long haul.

11-Embracing Food Variety and Culinary Exploration:

While the ketogenic diet emphasizes certain food groups, it's important to embrace food variety and culinary exploration within the confines of the diet. Explore new recipes, experiment with different ingredients and flavors, and challenge yourself to try new foods.

This not only keeps your meals exciting and enjoyable but also ensures you obtain a wide range of nutrients from different sources.

Incorporating a diverse array of foods helps to prevent dietary monotony and increases the sustainability of the ketogenic lifestyle.

12-Periodic Assessments and Adjustments:

As your body and health evolve, periodic assessments and adjustments to your ketogenic approach become necessary.

Regularly evaluate your goals, monitor your progress, and assess how your body is responding to the ketogenic lifestyle.

Consider consulting with a healthcare professional or registered dietitian experienced in ketogenic nutrition to fine-tune your approach.

By staying attentive and making necessary adjustments, you can optimize your ketogenic journey for continued success.

13-Emphasizing Whole Foods and Quality Ingredients:

To sustain long-term success on the ketogenic journey, prioritize whole, unprocessed foods and quality ingredients.

Choose organic, pasture-raised meats, wild-caught fish, and organic, locally sourced vegetables whenever possible.

Opt for healthy fats from sources like avocados, nuts, seeds, and cold-pressed oils. Minimize your consumption of processed and refined foods, which can be high in additives, preservatives, and unhealthy fats.

By nourishing your body with high-quality ingredients, you provide the essential nutrients needed for optimal health and well-being.

14-Embracing a Growth Mindset:

Adopting a growth mindset is crucial for sustaining long-term success.

Embrace the belief that your abilities, knowledge, and habits can continually evolve and improve.

View setbacks and challenges as opportunities for learning and growth rather than failures.

Cultivate resilience, perseverance, and a positive attitude as you navigate the ups and downs of your ketogenic journey.

By embracing a growth mindset, you can overcome obstacles, adapt to changes, and sustain your progress for years to come.

This Chapter has provided valuable strategies for sustaining long-term success on your ketogenic journey. By practicing mindful eating, engaging in regular physical activity, nurturing a positive mindset, finding balance and flexibility, continuing to learn and grow, tracking and monitoring progress, cultivating a supportive environment, celebrating non-scale victories, and embracing self-care and stress management, you can establish a sustainable approach to the ketogenic lifestyle.

Remember that sustained success is not just about reaching a specific goal but about creating a lifelong commitment to your health and well-being.

With dedication and perseverance, you can enjoy the long-term benefits of the ketogenic journey.

Chapter 11

Navigating Social Situations and Maintaining Ketogenic Success

In this chapter, we will explore strategies for navigating social situations while maintaining your ketogenic success.

Social events, dining out, and peer pressure can present challenges to adhering to the ketogenic lifestyle.

However, with the right mindset and preparation, you can stay committed to your health goals while still enjoying social interactions and gatherings.

1-Communicating Your Dietary Needs:

One of the first steps in navigating social situations is effectively communicating your dietary needs to others.

Let your friends, family, and colleagues know about your commitment to the ketogenic lifestyle and the reasons behind it.

Explain that you're focusing on your health and well-being and seek their understanding and support.

When attending events or gatherings, consider reaching out to the host in advance to discuss your dietary requirements and explore possible options.

2-Bringing Your Keto-Friendly Dish:

If you're uncertain about the food options available at a social gathering, consider bringing a keto-friendly dish to share.

This not only ensures that you have a suitable choice to enjoy but also introduces others to delicious and nutritious keto recipes.

Consider dishes such as a vegetable platter with a keto-friendly dip, a salad with low-carb dressings, or a flavorful meat dish.

By contributing to the spread, you're providing yourself and others with a healthier alternative.

3-Making Informed Menu Choices:

When dining out, it's essential to make informed menu choices that align with your ketogenic lifestyle.

Research restaurants in advance and review their menus online.

Look for dishes that feature high-quality proteins, healthy fats, and non-starchy vegetables.

Be mindful of hidden sources of carbohydrates, such as sauces, dressings, or marinades, and ask for modifications or substitutions as needed.

Don't be afraid to communicate your dietary preferences to the waitstaff, who are often willing to accommodate special requests.

4-Prioritizing Protein and Filling Vegetables:

In social situations, focus on prioritizing protein and filling vegetables to create a satisfying and nutritious meal.

Lean proteins, such as grilled chicken, fish, or steak, are excellent choices.

Non-starchy vegetables, such as leafy greens, broccoli, cauliflower, or asparagus, provide essential nutrients and fiber while keeping your carbohydrate intake in check. Fill your plate with these nutritious options to support your ketogenic goals.

5-Navigating Alcohol and Beverages:

Alcohol and sugary beverages can pose challenges to ketogenic success.

Alcoholic beverages often contain carbohydrates, which can affect ketosis and hinder progress.

Opt for spirits like vodka, gin, or tequila, and pair them with sugar-free mixers or soda water.

Be mindful of your alcohol consumption, as it can lower inhibitions and lead to impulsive food choices. Alternatively, choose non-alcoholic beverages like sparkling water with lemon or herbal tea to stay hydrated and refreshed.

6-Handling Peer Pressure and Social Judgment:

It's common to encounter peer pressure or social judgment when following a specific dietary approach.

Stay confident in your choices and remember your reasons for embracing the ketogenic lifestyle.

Educate others about the health benefits you've experienced and emphasize that everyone's dietary needs and preferences differ.

Surround yourself with a supportive community of like-minded individuals who understand and appreciate your commitment.

7-Developing Coping Strategies:

Developing coping strategies can help you navigate challenging social situations successfully.

Practice saying "no" politely but firmly when offered foods that don't align with your dietary goals.

Focus on the social aspects of the gathering rather than solely on the food.

Engage in conversation, enjoy the company of others, and shift your attention away from the food offerings.

Additionally, having a plan in place, such as pre-eating a keto-friendly meal or carrying a keto snack, can help you resist temptation and make healthier choices.

8-Balancing Indulgences:

Maintaining balance is key when faced with indulgent foods or treats in social situations.

While it's essential to stay committed to your health goals, occasional indulgences can be part of a sustainable ketogenic lifestyle.

If you decide to indulge, do so mindfully and in moderation.

Be selective about your choices and savor the flavors and textures.

Remember that one indulgence does not define your overall progress, and you can get back on track with your ketogenic approach.

9-Building a Supportive Network:

Having a supportive network is essential when navigating social situations while maintaining your ketogenic success.

Surround yourself with individuals who understand and respect your dietary choices.

Seek out online communities, social media groups, or local meetup groups that are focused on the ketogenic lifestyle.

Engaging with like-minded individuals can provide encouragement, advice, and a sense of belonging.

Additionally, consider involving friends and family in your journey, educating them about the ketogenic lifestyle, and enlisting their support.

10-Planning for Social Events:

Planning is crucial for successfully navigating social events.

Before attending an event, find out as much as possible about the food options available. If necessary, contact the host or organizer to discuss your dietary needs and inquire about any potential accommodations.

Consider eating a small keto-friendly meal or snack before the event to help you resist tempting high-carb options.

By planning, you can ensure you have suitable choices and reduce the stress associated with uncertain food situations.

11-Educating Yourself and Others:

Education plays a vital role in navigating social situations.

Continually educate yourself about the ketogenic lifestyle, its benefits, and the science behind it.

This knowledge will not only help you stay committed to your goals but also enable you to explain your choices to others clearly and confidently.

Be prepared to answer questions about the ketogenic diet, dispel misconceptions, and share your personal experiences.

By educating yourself and others, you can foster understanding and promote a supportive environment.

12-Developing Resilience and Confidence:

Developing resilience and confidence is essential when faced with social challenges.

Embrace the fact that your dietary choices are personal and that your health and well-being are top priorities.

Believe in the value of your commitment and the positive impact it has on your life.

Stay resilient in the face of criticism or judgment, knowing that you are making choices that align with your goals and values.

By building confidence and resilience, you can navigate social situations with greater ease and conviction.

13-Seeking Alternative Social Activities:

Socializing doesn't always have to revolve around food. Seek out alternative activities that allow you to connect with others while maintaining your ketogenic lifestyle.

Consider hosting a keto-friendly potluck or gathering where everyone can enjoy delicious, healthy dishes.

Explore outdoor activities, fitness classes, or group hobbies that align with your interests.

By shifting the focus away from food-centered gatherings, you can still enjoy social interactions while staying true to your health goals.

14-Practicing Self-Compassion:

Throughout your ketogenic journey, it's essential to practice self-compassion, especially in social situations.

If you find yourself deviating from your plan or making less-than-ideal choices, avoid self-judgment and instead focus on self-care and self-encouragement.

Remember that setbacks are normal, and every day is an opportunity to make healthier choices.

Be kind to yourself, learn from the experience, and recommit to your ketogenic lifestyle with a renewed sense of determination.

This Chapter has provided detailed strategies for navigating social situations while maintaining your ketogenic success.

By effectively communicating your dietary needs, bringing keto-friendly dishes, making informed menu choices, prioritizing protein and vegetables, navigating alcohol and beverages, handling peer pressure, developing coping strategies, balancing indulgences, building a supportive network, planning for social events, educating yourself and others, developing resilience and confidence, seeking alternative social activities, and practicing self-compassion, you can navigate social situations with ease and continue to thrive on your ketogenic journey.

Remember, the key is to prioritize your health goals while still enjoying meaningful connections and social interactions. With these strategies in place, you can successfully maintain your ketogenic success and live a fulfilling and balanced life.

Chapter 12

Overcoming Plateaus and Challenges on the Ketogenic Journey

In this chapter, we will explore strategies for overcoming plateaus and challenges that may arise during your ketogenic journey.

Plateaus, where weight loss or other health benefits stall, can be frustrating, and it's essential to have strategies in place to overcome them. Additionally, we will address common challenges and obstacles that you may encounter on your ketogenic journey and provide practical solutions to help you stay on track.

1-Understanding Plateaus:

Plateaus are a common occurrence during any weight loss or health transformation journey, including the ketogenic diet.

It's important to understand that plateaus are a natural part of the process and often indicate that your body is adjusting and adapting to the changes. Recognize that weight loss is not linear and that your body may need time to recalibrate before continuing to progress.

By reframing plateaus as temporary setbacks rather than failures, you can approach them with a more positive mindset.

2-Reassessing Your Approach:

When facing a plateau, it's crucial to reassess your approach and identify any potential areas for improvement.

Take a closer look at your macronutrient intake, portion sizes, and overall calorie consumption.

Ensure that you are accurately tracking your food intake and not unknowingly consuming more carbohydrates or calories than intended.

Consider consulting with a registered dietitian or healthcare professional with expertise in the ketogenic diet to help you review your approach and make necessary adjustments.

3-Fine-Tuning Macros and Caloric Intake:

Fine-tuning your macronutrient ratios and caloric intake can be beneficial for breaking through plateaus.

Gradually adjust your macronutrient ratios, such as increasing your fat intake or reducing your protein intake, to find the optimal balance for your body.

Experiment with calorie cycling, where you alternate between higher and lower calorie days, to keep your metabolism stimulated.

These adjustments can help overcome plateaus and stimulate further progress on your ketogenic journey.

4-Incorporating Intermittent Fasting:

Intermittent fasting is a powerful tool that can be utilized to overcome plateaus and stimulate weight loss on the ketogenic diet.

By implementing periods of fasting, you create a favorable environment for fat-burning and metabolic flexibility.

Consider incorporating different fasting protocols, such as 16:8 (16 hours of fasting, 8 hours of eating) or alternate-day fasting, and find the approach that works best for you.

However, it's important to approach fasting with caution and consult with a healthcare professional if you have any underlying health conditions.

5-Prioritizing Nutrient Density:

Nutrient density plays a crucial role in overall health and can be instrumental in overcoming plateaus.

Focus on incorporating a wide variety of nutrient-dense foods into your ketogenic diet, such as leafy greens, cruciferous vegetables, colorful berries, and high-quality proteins.

These foods provide essential vitamins, minerals, and antioxidants, which support optimal metabolic function and overall well-being.

By prioritizing nutrient density, you ensure that your body is receiving the necessary fuel to break through plateaus and thrive.

6-Incorporating Physical Activity:

Physical activity is not only beneficial for weight management but also for breaking through plateaus and enhancing overall health.

Consider incorporating both aerobic exercises, such as brisk walking or cycling, and strength training exercises to promote fat burning, preserve lean muscle mass, and boost your metabolism.

Engage in activities that you enjoy and that align with your fitness level.

Consult with a healthcare professional or a qualified fitness trainer to design an exercise plan tailored to your specific needs.

7-Managing Stress and Sleep:

Stress and inadequate sleep can hinder progress on your ketogenic journey.

Elevated stress levels can lead to hormonal imbalances and hinder fat loss, while poor sleep can disrupt metabolic processes.

Prioritize stress management techniques such as meditation, deep breathing exercises, or engaging in hobbies and activities that promote relaxation.

Aim for a consistent sleep schedule and create a sleep-friendly environment to ensure you're getting adequate rest.

By managing stress and optimizing sleep, you support your body's ability to overcome plateaus and achieve optimal health.

8-Seeking Support and Accountability:

During challenging times, seeking support and accountability can make a significant difference in staying motivated and overcoming plateaus.

Connect with others who are on a similar ketogenic journey through online communities, local support groups, or wellness programs.

Share your challenges, celebrate successes, and learn from others' experiences.

Consider partnering with a friend or family member to hold each other accountable and provide mutual support.

The encouragement and camaraderie found in a supportive community can help you push through plateaus and stay committed to your goals.

9-Practicing Mindful Eating:

Mindful eating involves paying attention to the sensory experience of eating and being fully present at the moment.

By practicing mindful eating, you can develop a greater awareness of your body's hunger and fullness cues.

This can help you avoid overeating and make more conscious food choices.

When faced with a plateau, incorporate mindful eating practices into your daily routine.

Slow down while eating, savor each bite, and tune in to the signals your body is sending.

This mindful approach can help you better understand your body's needs and make adjustments accordingly.

10-Tracking Non-Scale Victories:

While weight loss is often a primary focus on the ketogenic journey, it's important to recognize and celebrate non-scale victories.

Plateaus may not always reflect changes on the scale, but other positive changes could be occurring. Track and celebrate improvements in energy levels, mental clarity, improved sleep quality, clothes fitting better, increased strength or endurance during physical activity, or improvements in biomarkers like blood pressure or cholesterol levels.

By shifting your focus beyond the number on the scale, you can maintain motivation and continue to see progress.

11-Embracing a Growth Mindset:

A growth mindset is the belief that challenges and setbacks are opportunities for growth and learning. Adopting a growth mindset can be particularly helpful when facing plateaus and challenges on your ketogenic journey.

Instead of viewing plateaus as failures, see them as opportunities to learn more about your body and make necessary adjustments.

Embrace the journey as a process of self-discovery and continuous improvement.

By maintaining a positive and growth-oriented mindset, you can stay resilient, learn from setbacks, and keep moving forward.

12-Celebrating Progress and Gratitude:

Take time to acknowledge and celebrate the progress you have made on your ketogenic journey.

Reflect on how far you have come, the positive changes you have experienced, and the lessons you have learned. Practice gratitude for your body's resilience, your commitment to your health, and the support you have received along the way.

By cultivating a mindset of gratitude and celebrating even the smallest victories, you can stay motivated, maintain perspective, and overcome challenges with resilience and positivity.

13-Seeking Professional Guidance:

If you find yourself consistently struggling with plateaus or facing significant challenges on your ketogenic journey, don't hesitate to seek professional guidance.

Consulting with a registered dietitian, nutritionist, or healthcare professional with expertise in ketogenic diets can provide personalized guidance, support, and recommendations based on your specific needs.

They can help identify potential underlying factors contributing to plateaus and offer tailored strategies to overcome them.

Remember, seeking professional guidance is an investment in your health and can provide valuable insights to help you break through barriers.

This Chapter has explored various strategies for overcoming plateaus and challenges on the ketogenic journey.

By practicing mindful eating, tracking non-scale victories, embracing a growth mindset, celebrating progress and gratitude, and seeking professional guidance when needed, you can navigate through plateaus and maintain long-term success on your ketogenic journey.

Remember, the path to optimal health is not always linear, and challenges are an opportunity for growth. With persistence, adaptability, and the right strategies in place, you can overcome plateaus and continue progressing toward your health goals.

Chapter 13

Sustaining Long-Term Success on the Ketogenic Journey

In this chapter, we will delve into strategies for sustaining long-term success on the ketogenic journey. While starting a ketogenic diet can yield significant benefits, maintaining the lifestyle, in the long run, requires consistency, commitment, and the ability to navigate potential pitfalls.

This chapter will provide you with the tools and knowledge to sustain your progress, optimize your health, and make the ketogenic lifestyle a lifelong journey.

1-Establishing a Sustainable Routine:

Creating a sustainable routine is crucial for long-term success on the ketogenic journey.

Develop a meal plan that incorporates a variety of delicious and nutrient-dense foods while adhering to your macronutrient goals.

Plan and prep your meals ahead of time to avoid relying on convenient but high-carb options.

Incorporate regular physical activity into your routine, finding activities that you enjoy and that fit your lifestyle.

By establishing a sustainable routine, you can easily adhere to your ketogenic lifestyle and make it a seamless part of your daily life.

2-Expanding Your Culinary Repertoire:

Maintaining long-term success on the ketogenic journey doesn't mean sacrificing flavor or variety in your meals. Embrace the opportunity to expand your culinary repertoire by experimenting with new recipes, flavors, and cooking techniques.

Explore keto-friendly cookbooks, online resources, and social media platforms dedicated to ketogenic recipes.

By continuously introducing new and exciting dishes into your diet, you can prevent food monotony, keep your taste buds satisfied, and stay motivated to stick with your ketogenic lifestyle.

3-Practicing Intuitive Eating:

Intuitive eating involves listening to your body's hunger and fullness cues, and it can be a valuable tool for sustaining long-term success on the ketogenic journey.

Instead of relying solely on external guidelines and strict meal plans, tune in to your body's natural signals.

Eat when you're hungry and stop when you're satisfied, paying attention to how different foods make you feel.

Trust your body's wisdom to guide your food choices, making adjustments as necessary.

By practicing intuitive eating, you can cultivate a healthy and balanced relationship with food while maintaining your ketogenic goals.

4-Prioritizing Whole Foods:

Whole foods should form the foundation of your ketogenic diet for optimal health and sustainability.

Focus on incorporating whole, minimally processed foods such as vegetables, fruits in moderation, lean proteins, healthy fats, and nuts and seeds.

These foods provide essential nutrients, fiber, and phytochemicals that support overall well-being.

Minimize your intake of processed and packaged keto-friendly products, which may contain hidden sugars, artificial additives, or unhealthy fats.

By prioritizing whole foods, you nourish your body with the nutrients it needs for sustained health and vitality.

5-Monitoring and Adjusting as Needed:

Regular monitoring and self-assessment are crucial for sustaining long-term success on the ketogenic journey.

Keep track of your progress, including weight, body measurements, energy levels, and overall well-being.

Consider monitoring ketone levels using blood, urine, or breath tests to ensure you're in a state of ketosis.

Be open to making adjustments as needed based on your personal goals and health markers.

Consult with a healthcare professional or registered dietitian with expertise in the ketogenic diet to guide you in assessing and adjusting your approach.

6-Cultivating a Supportive Environment:

Surrounding yourself with a supportive environment can significantly impact your long-term success on the ketogenic journey.

Engage with a community of individuals who share your goals and values, whether through online forums, local support groups, or social media networks.

Seek support from friends and family members who understand and respect your dietary choices.

Communicate your needs and preferences to those around you, and encourage their support.

By cultivating a supportive environment, you create a foundation for success and accountability.

7-Managing Social and Emotional Challenges:

Social and emotional challenges can arise when following a ketogenic lifestyle, especially in social situations or during times of stress.

Develop strategies to navigate these challenges effectively.

When dining out, research keto-friendly options beforehand, communicate your dietary preferences to the server or offer to bring a dish that aligns with your needs.

Find alternative ways to cope with stress or emotional triggers that don't involve food, such as engaging in physical activity, practicing mindfulness, or seeking support from loved ones.

By proactively managing social and emotional challenges, you can stay on track and maintain your ketogenic lifestyle.

8-Setting Realistic and Flexible Goals:

Setting realistic and flexible goals is essential for sustaining long-term success on the ketogenic journey.

Rather than solely focusing on a specific number on the scale, consider broader health-related goals such as improving energy levels, enhancing mental clarity, or reducing inflammation.

Set realistic expectations for your progress and allow for flexibility as your body adjusts to the ketogenic lifestyle.

Embrace the journey as a continuous process of growth and improvement, acknowledging that progress may vary from person to person.

By setting realistic and flexible goals, you can maintain motivation and stay committed for the long term.

9-Practicing Self-Care:

Self-care is vital for sustaining long-term success on the ketogenic journey.

Prioritize activities that promote relaxation, stress reduction, and overall well-being.

Engage in practices such as meditation, yoga, journaling, or spending time in nature.

Take breaks when needed and allow yourself moments of indulgence without feeling guilty.

Remember that self-care goes beyond just food choices and includes nurturing your mind, body, and spirit.

By prioritizing self-care, you create a foundation of self-love and holistic wellness that supports your ketogenic lifestyle.

10-Continuing Education and Learning:

Staying informed and continuing to educate yourself about the ketogenic diet is crucial for sustaining long-term success.

Keep up with the latest research, resources, and developments in the field of ketogenic nutrition.

Stay connected with reputable sources of information, such as scientific journals, books, podcasts, or websites run by trusted experts.

By continuously expanding your knowledge, you can deepen your understanding of the ketogenic lifestyle and make informed decisions about your dietary choices. Seek opportunities to learn and grow on your journey.

11-Practicing Mindset and Gratitude:

Maintaining a positive mindset and cultivating gratitude can greatly impact your long-term success on the ketogenic journey.

Practice daily affirmations, visualization, or gratitude exercises to reinforce a positive mindset.

Focus on the benefits and positive changes you've experienced in the ketogenic lifestyle, expressing gratitude for the transformation in your health and well-being.

Embrace challenges as opportunities for growth and learning.

By nurturing a positive mindset and cultivating gratitude, you foster a sense of empowerment and resilience that supports your sustained success.

12-Embracing Flexibility and Adaptability:

Life is dynamic, and circumstances may change over time. Embrace flexibility and adaptability as integral parts of your ketogenic journey.

Be open to adjusting your approach as needed, whether it's modifying your macronutrient ratios, exploring different meal plans, or trying new recipes.

Embrace the concept of metabolic flexibility, where your body can efficiently switch between fuel sources.

This flexibility allows you to navigate different situations, such as travel, special occasions, or lifestyle changes, while still adhering to the principles of the ketogenic lifestyle.

By embracing flexibility and adaptability, you can sustain your progress regardless of the challenges that come your way.

This Chapter has explored additional strategies for sustaining long-term success on the ketogenic journey. By setting realistic and flexible goals, practicing self-care, continuing education, and learning, nurturing a positive mindset and gratitude, and embracing flexibility and adaptability, you can thrive on your ketogenic journey for years to come.

Remember that sustaining success is a lifelong commitment, and it requires ongoing effort and dedication.

With these strategies in place, you can cultivate a sustainable and fulfilling ketogenic lifestyle that supports your optimal health and well-being.

Chapter 14

Troubleshooting Common Challenges on the Ketogenic Journey

In this chapter, we will address common challenges that individuals may encounter on their ketogenic journey and provide effective strategies for troubleshooting and overcoming them.

From managing keto flu symptoms to addressing cravings and dealing with social pressures, this chapter will equip you with the knowledge and tools to navigate through potential roadblocks and maintain your progress toward optimal health.

1-Managing Keto Flu Symptoms:

The keto flu is a collection of symptoms that some individuals may experience when transitioning into a ketogenic diet.

These symptoms can include fatigue, headache, dizziness, irritability, and sugar cravings.

To manage keto flu symptoms, ensure you are properly hydrated and replenish electrolytes by consuming foods rich in sodium, potassium, and magnesium or by using electrolyte supplements.

Gradually reduce your carbohydrate intake instead of making an abrupt shift to help your body adapt more smoothly.

Be patient, as these symptoms are usually temporary and will resolve as your body becomes keto-adapted.

2-Dealing with Cravings:

Cravings for high-carbohydrate foods can be a challenge on the ketogenic journey.

To address cravings, it's essential to identify the underlying causes.

Are you truly hungry, or are you experiencing emotional or habitual cravings? If hunger is the issue, ensure you are consuming enough healthy fats and protein to keep you satiated.

If emotional or habitual cravings arise, find alternative activities such as engaging in a hobby, going for a walk, or practicing mindfulness techniques to distract yourself.

You can also explore keto-friendly substitutes for your favorite high-carb foods to satisfy cravings without derailing your progress.

3-Overcoming Weight Loss Plateaus:

Weight loss plateaus are a common occurrence on any weight loss journey, including the ketogenic diet.

To overcome plateaus, reassess your dietary habits and ensure you are still in a calorie deficit.

Consider adjusting your macronutrient ratios or experimenting with intermittent fasting to jumpstart your metabolism. Incorporating resistance training and other forms of physical activity can also help rev up your metabolism and break through plateaus.

Stay consistent with your ketogenic lifestyle and be patient, as weight loss progress can vary from person to person.

4-Navigating Social Pressures:

Social situations can present challenges on the ketogenic journey, as others may not understand or support your dietary choices.

To navigate social pressures, communicate your dietary needs and goals to your friends, family, and social circle.

Offer to bring a keto-friendly dish to gatherings to ensure you have options available.

Educate others about the benefits of the ketogenic lifestyle and the science behind it.

Remember to prioritize your health and well-being, and don't feel compelled to compromise your goals due to external pressures.

Surround yourself with a supportive community or find online support groups where you can connect with like-minded individuals who understand your journey.

5-Addressing Digestive Issues:

Some individuals may experience digestive issues when starting a ketogenic diet.

This can include constipation, diarrhea, or changes in bowel movements.

To address digestive issues, ensure you are consuming an adequate amount of fiber from non-starchy vegetables, nuts, and seeds.

Hydration is crucial, so drink plenty of water throughout the day.

Consider incorporating probiotic-rich foods such as sauerkraut, kimchi, or kefir to promote a healthy gut microbiome. If issues persist, consult with a healthcare professional to rule out any underlying medical conditions or explore potential dietary adjustments.

6-Managing Travel and Dining Out:

Traveling or dining out while following a ketogenic lifestyle can be challenging but not impossible.

Plan by researching keto-friendly restaurants or menu options at your travel destination.

Pack keto-friendly snacks for when you're on the go.

Be clear and assertive when communicating your dietary needs to waitstaff or hosts.

Opt for protein-rich dishes with healthy fats and non-starchy vegetables.

Remember that it's okay to make modifications or substitutions to suit your dietary requirements.

By preparing and being proactive, you can enjoy your travels or dining experiences while staying true to your ketogenic goals.

7-Handling Emotional Eating:

Emotional eating is a common challenge that can arise on any dietary journey, including the ketogenic diet.

It's important to recognize the triggers and emotions that lead to emotional eating and develop alternative coping mechanisms.

Engage in activities that help reduce stress and manage emotions, such as practicing meditation, journaling, or seeking support from loved ones.

Build a strong support system that can provide encouragement and understanding during challenging times.

Additionally, practicing mindful eating can help you become more aware of your hunger and satiety cues, allowing you to make conscious food choices instead of turning to emotional eating.

8-Balancing Social Life and Ketogenic Lifestyle:

Maintaining a social life while following a ketogenic lifestyle may require some adjustments, but it is entirely possible.

When attending social events or gatherings, plan by eating a satisfying and keto-friendly meal beforehand. Focus on socializing and enjoying the company of others rather than solely focusing on the food.

Look for keto-friendly options or make modifications when possible, and don't be afraid to communicate your dietary needs to hosts or friends.

Remember that your health and well-being are important, and making choices aligned with your ketogenic lifestyle doesn't mean sacrificing social connections or enjoyment.

9-Staying Motivated:

Sustaining motivation is key to long-term success on the ketogenic journey.

Find sources of inspiration that resonate with you, such as success stories, educational resources, or engaging with a supportive community.

Set short-term goals that are achievable and track your progress along the way.

Celebrate milestones and non-scale victories to stay motivated beyond just the number on the scale.

Keep a journal to reflect on your journey, including the positive changes you've experienced physically, mentally, and emotionally.

Surround yourself with visual reminders of your goals, such as affirmations or images that represent your desired outcomes.

Remember that motivation may ebb and flow, but with consistent effort and a supportive mindset, you can maintain long-term success.

10-Seeking Professional Guidance:

If you encounter persistent challenges or require personalized support, seeking guidance from healthcare professionals or registered dietitians with expertise in the ketogenic diet can be immensely valuable.

They can provide individualized recommendations, address specific concerns, and help tailor your ketogenic journey to your unique needs.

A professional can assess your progress, guide you in troubleshooting challenges, and provide evidence-based advice to optimize your health and well-being.

This Chapter has explored various common challenges that individuals may encounter on their ketogenic journey and provided effective strategies for troubleshooting and overcoming them.

By managing keto flu symptoms, dealing with cravings, overcoming weight loss plateaus, navigating social pressures, addressing digestive issues, managing travel and dining out, handling emotional eating, balancing social life, staying motivated, and seeking professional guidance when needed, you can overcome obstacles and maintain your progress on the ketogenic path.

Remember that the journey is a continuous learning process, and with patience, resilience, and a positive mindset, you can successfully overcome challenges and achieve sustainable success on your ketogenic journey.

Chapter 15

Sustainable Ketogenic Living for Long-Term Health

We will explore the principles and practices of sustainable ketogenic living for long-term health.

Transitioning to a ketogenic lifestyle is not just about achieving short-term results; it's about embracing a way of life that promotes overall well-being, metabolic flexibility, and optimal health.

By integrating sustainable habits into your daily routine, you can ensure that the benefits of the ketogenic diet continue to enhance your life for years to come.

1-Emphasizing Whole Foods:

A cornerstone of sustainable ketogenic living is the emphasis on whole, nutrient-dense foods.

Focus on consuming a variety of non-starchy vegetables, high-quality protein sources, healthy fats, nuts, seeds, and low-sugar fruits.

Opt for organic, locally sourced, and minimally processed foods whenever possible.

Whole foods provide essential nutrients, fiber, and phytochemicals that support optimal health and contribute to sustained well-being.

2-Mindful Eating and Intuitive Listening:

Practice mindful eating to cultivate a deeper connection with your body and its nutritional needs.

Slow down and savor each bite, paying attention to the flavors, textures, and sensations of the food.

Eat when you are hungry and stop when you are satisfied, practicing intuitive listening to your body's signals.

Avoid distractions such as screens or multitasking during meals, allowing yourself to fully engage with the eating experience.

By practicing mindful eating and intuitive listening, you can develop a more balanced and sustainable relationship with food.

3-Prioritizing Sleep and Stress Management:

Quality sleep and effective stress management are crucial for sustainable ketogenic living.

Prioritize getting adequate restful sleep by establishing a consistent sleep schedule, creating a conducive sleep environment, and practicing relaxation techniques before bed.

Incorporate stress management practices such as meditation, yoga, deep breathing exercises, or engaging in hobbies that bring joy and relaxation.

Chronic stress and insufficient sleep can disrupt hormonal balance, hinder weight loss efforts, and impact overall well-being.

By prioritizing sleep and stress management, you support the body's healing processes and optimize the benefits of the ketogenic lifestyle.

4-Regular Physical Activity:

Regular physical activity is an essential component of sustainable ketogenic living.

Engage in activities that you enjoy and that align with your fitness level and preferences.

Incorporate a combination of cardiovascular exercise, strength training, and flexibility exercises into your routine.

Regular physical activity helps maintain muscle mass, supports healthy metabolism, improves cardiovascular health, enhances mood, and contributes to long-term weight management.

Find ways to incorporate movement into your daily life, such as walking or biking instead of driving, taking the stairs instead of the elevator, or participating in recreational sports.

Aim for consistency rather than perfection and prioritize finding joy in movement.

5-Continual Learning and Growth:

Sustainable ketogenic living involves a commitment to continual learning and growth.

Stay informed about the latest research and developments in the field of ketogenic nutrition.

Explore new recipes, cooking techniques, and meal-planning strategies to expand your culinary repertoire.

Seek out educational resources, books, podcasts, or online communities that provide support, motivation, and inspiration.

Embrace the journey as a lifelong process of self-discovery, growth, and refinement.

By continuously learning and growing, you can adapt to new information, refine your practices, and optimize your ketogenic lifestyle.

6-Cultivating Social Support:

Building a strong support system is crucial for sustaining a ketogenic lifestyle.

Surround yourself with individuals who understand and support your dietary choices.

Seek out like-minded individuals in your community or online platforms who share similar health goals.

Engage in group activities or join local ketogenic support groups where you can connect with others, exchange ideas, and share experiences.

Having a supportive network can provide encouragement, accountability, and motivation on your sustainable ketogenic journey.

7-Regular Monitoring and Adjustments:

To maintain long-term success, it's important to regularly monitor and assess your progress.

Keep track of key indicators such as weight, body measurements, blood glucose levels, ketone levels, and energy levels.

This monitoring allows you to identify any potential imbalances or areas for improvement.

Adjust your macronutrient ratios, caloric intake, or exercise routine as needed to optimize your results.

Regular check-ins with healthcare professionals or registered dietitians can provide valuable guidance and ensure you are on track for long-term success.

8-Incorporating Flexibility:

While the ketogenic lifestyle emphasizes certain dietary guidelines, it's essential to incorporate flexibility to ensure long-term sustainability.

Allow for occasional deviations or modifications to suit special occasions, travel, or social events.

Experiment with cyclical ketogenic approaches or targeted ketogenic strategies if they align with your goals and preferences.

Remember that sustainability is about finding a balance that works for you, allowing for the enjoyment of food and life while maintaining the principles of a ketogenic lifestyle.

9-Practicing Self-Compassion:

As you embark on the journey of sustainable ketogenic living, it's important to practice self-compassion and embrace a positive mindset.

Understand that setbacks and challenges may occur, but they are opportunities for growth and learning.

Be kind to yourself and avoid self-judgment or criticism. Celebrate your successes, both big and small, and acknowledge the progress you've made.

Embrace self-care practices that nourish your mind, body, and soul, such as engaging in hobbies, practicing self-reflection, and seeking moments of joy and gratitude.

10-Embracing Long-Term Health Benefits:

Sustainable ketogenic living goes beyond weight loss and short-term results.

Embrace the long-term health benefits that come with this lifestyle.

Improved insulin sensitivity, blood sugar regulation, cardiovascular health, mental clarity, and sustained energy levels are just a few of the many benefits.

Remember that sustainable health is a holistic approach that encompasses not only nutrition but also emotional well-being, stress management, sleep, and physical activity.

Embrace the journey as an investment in your long-term health and overall quality of life.

This Chapter has explored the principles and practices of sustainable ketogenic living for long-term health.

By incorporating whole foods, practicing mindful eating, prioritizing sleep and stress management, engaging in regular physical activity, cultivating social support, monitoring progress, embracing flexibility, practicing self-compassion, and embracing the long-term health benefits, you can lead a sustainable and fulfilling ketogenic lifestyle.

Remember that sustainable living is a continuous process of self-discovery, self-care, and growth.

With dedication, flexibility, and a positive mindset, you can enjoy the lifelong benefits of the ketogenic diet while embracing a well-rounded and vibrant life.

Printed in Great Britain
by Amazon